Say Goodbye to Panic Attacks

The Wasted Years

*In proud and loving memory
of my dearest Gran*

Say Goodbye to Panic Attacks

The Wasted Years

Deanna Peedell

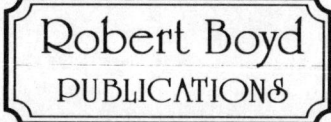
Robert Boyd PUBLICATIONS

Published by
Robert Boyd Publications
260 Colwell Drive
Witney, Oxfordshire OX8 7LW

Copyright © Deanna Peedell

First Published 1996

ISBN: 1 899536 08 6

Printed and bound by Oxuniprint, Walton Street, Oxford, OX2 6DP

Contents

Acknowledgements	6
Foreword	7
Preface	9
Introduction	11
1. My early years	13
2. The panic attacks begin	16
3. More attacks	20
4. The boys	24
5. Back to work	27
6. The medical establishment	30
7. Dr. Ritchie and the diet	34
8. Disappointing dates	42
9. St. Giles Fair revisited	45
10. The exclusion diet	47
11. Footnote	70
12. Appendix	71

Acknowledgements

Among the many people to whom I must express my gratitude for so many kindnesses, the principal ones must be my husband, Alan, and my sons, Derek and Clive. Over the years, they have had to endure my condition and this they have done with patience and understanding. I am only sorry that they have had to wait for so long to see any improvement.

Mr. Ken Halsey helped me to set out my first synopsis of the book. I am particularly grateful to certain members of the medical profession, especially to Dr. J. Ritchie for giving me relief from panic attacks, Dr. L.W. Blazewicz for his help and encouragement over many years, Dr. J.O. Hunter of Addenbrookes Hospital for permission to reproduce details of the exclusion diet, and the doctors at the Botley (Oxford) Medical Centre.

Mrs. Carol Phipps, despite having had major cancer surgery herself, has found the time to help me through those periods when I doubted that this volume would ever appear and Mr. Geoff Parkinson produced the final text from the original draft.

A special word of thanks is due to Blondine L. Reddick of Longwood, Florida, U.S.A. for her precious time and the encouragement she has provided to help me see the book through to publication.

Foreword

Dr. L.W. Blazewicz, M.A., M.R.C.P, M.R.C.G.P

The occurrence of acute overwhelming dread is a most debilitating experience. Such panic attacks are often accompanied by an explosion of autonomic activity with dizziness, sweating, palpitations, etc., which can last from a matter of a few minutes to several hours and leave the victim drained and weak.

This is the story of Deanna Peedell, an intelligent, alert, capable lady whose life became a nightmare of panic attacks and disabling asthma. She was subjected to multidisciplinary assessments and investigations seeking an organic aetiology, until finally a miraculous transformation occurred when she observed food intolerance emerging as a significant precipitating factor. She often felt guilt, shame and failure but she never gave up hope. Her observed response to exclusions and challenge was so exquisite that the results were clearly quite beyond the scope of pure chance.

She hopes her experiences of exclusion, substitutions and challenge will help others gain insight into their problems. Her progress from panic attacks, nasal allergies, to asthma suggests that early recognition and treatment may prevent full blown atopy syndrome occurring.

She has realised the importance of self-control, relaxation and diet. Her personal experiences will help you and will demonstrate that no hurdles in life are insurmountable.

April 1996

Preface

It was not my aim, when I began this book, to write an autobiography, nor have I done so. However, for two reasons I felt that it was necessary to include a short account of some of those aspects of my life which have been affected by my panic attacks. The first of these is to allow fellow sufferers to compare their experiences with mine and thus draw any parallels they feel might be useful to them in deciding whether to try for themselves the dietary approach to relief. The second reason is to help any non-sufferer who may happen to read these pages to obtain some idea of what we sufferers go through and so, perhaps, be more understanding of another member of the family.

In describing my experiences, I hope that I do not give the impression that I consider the use of tranquilisers to be universally bad. That is certainly not my position. I am, for example, from time to time prescribed antibiotics because of my asthma and for reducing the size of nasal polyps before their surgical removal and tranquilisers are effective in controlling the side effects of the steroids. Under those conditions I am pleased to use them.

The principal aims in producing the book, of course, are to show how the condition can be controlled by diet, to give an indication of how I arrived at the knowledge of what foods I must avoid, and, finally, to present a selection of recipes which I hope will demonstrate that a restricted diet need not be a dull one.

Since it became known that I was working on this volume, I have been encouraged by the number of sufferers from many different parts of the world, notably Australia, New Zealand, the United States and Sweden, who have taken the trouble to contact me enquiring about progress. If nothing else, it has shown me that there is a real need for such a book. In the meantime, I hope that I have been able to help some of the enquirers by telephone and letter and that their problems have been alleviated to some extent while waiting for the book to appear.

A Swedish lady who telephoned recently told me that she regards all the thirty-odd years she has suffered from panic attacks as having been wasted. I trust this volume will help her and many more panic attack victims to end their own wasted years.

Introduction

Dr. Clive Peedell, B.M.

It is sometimes very hard as a child to understand how your parents think and behave. In the case of my mother it was particularly so.

I had no idea that she suffered from panic attacks and agoraphobia until I was a teenager. With the benefit of hindsight, I can remember numerous occasions on which Mum demonstrated classic agoraphobic symptoms and behaviour. For example, my brother and I were baffled as children when she would take us out in the car to go swimming but before we ever got to the pool would turn the car round and drive home again, complaining of suddenly feeling unwell. She would reach into the glove compartment for her bottle of tablets and frantically swallow a couple whilst Derek and I cried in the back of the car, distraught that we would not be swimming that day. The tears soon subsided, however, once we reached home and, when she was feeling better, she gave us a bag of sweets each by way of apology. I have to say that, to this day, my teeth are pretty awful!

We also noticed that at school functions and on visits to the cinema Mum would always sit as close as she possibly could to the exit. Often she would fall asleep during a film, which might have been a consequence of taking her tablets. I now wonder how she managed to drive us home safely afterwards.

The worst memories, though, were the nocturnal stomach pains and panic attacks. I had more than a few sleepless nights as Mum rushed downstairs in a drenching sweat for her tablets followed by Dad who would be there to reassure her.

It amazes me now that, despite all the difficulties Mum encountered, Derek and I had a wonderful childhood. It was largely due to Mum's determination to do as many things as possible for us. She was able, for example, to take us to Belgium and Holland; certainly it was with the help of her Valium, but nevertheless she did it.

Only those who have experienced a panic attack could ever understand how difficult her life must have been. Now that I have qualified as a doctor and have a little more knowledge of the condition, I have the utmost respect for her courage and her perseverence to find the cure for her attacks which has enabled her to enrich her own life and those of the other members of her family.

1

My Early Years

I was born in Oxford during World War II. The post-war years were a difficult time for many people, but for me, at least when I was old enough to realise it, it seemed particularly so because I was illegitimate, a much more serious drawback for a young child in those days than it is now. My father was a Canadian soldier and we never met, although towards the end of his life we did have some contact by telephone.

My mother and I, together with other members of the extended family, lived with my grandmother in a large house on Walton Street and I attended the local school, St. Barnabas, where I suffered quite badly from the taunts of the other children.

And it was not only the children who made my life miserable. I used to attend a local ballet school run by Audrey Mallett and we were due to stage a dance programme at Exeter College. For my part in the Sailor's Hornpipe I had to have a sailor costume made and I vividly remember my grandmother sending me with the dress material to a local needlewoman. Initially the woman seemed ready to help, but when she realised who, or rather what, I was she remembered that she was overburdened with work and said she was unable to make the costume for me, and she lost no time in slamming the door in my face! Time was short but an aunt rallied round, cutting out and hand stitching the costume in one afternoon. I was, however, under strict instructions not to lift my arms nor kick my legs too high during the performance.

This was not an isolated incident. It was the sort of thing that happened all the time, but it was particularly bad at school. Children can be very cruel even if they do not always appreciate it at the time. Many years after leaving school and long after we were married, my husband, Alan, said to me,

'Some people gave you a pretty rough time when you were young, didn't they?'

They certainly did.

I am not suggesting that the sort of treatment I suffered when I was young had any connection with my later panic attacks but it did have a considerable influence on my character. It made me a fighter, someone who was determined to rise above all the troubles and make the best of my life. It was later to stand me in very good stead.

I went to St. Barnabas School from the time I was about five years old until I was fifteen, the normal school leaving age at that time. Alan had also been a pupil there but I have to admit that I did not immediately like him. His mother remembers me from those days as a pale-faced little girl surrounded by the smaller children of our family whom I had to take out and care for. She has told me that she used to hope that I would one day marry someone nice, little realising that the someone would be her own son!

My ambition while at school had been to work in an office and my grandmother, who was always very good to me, had paid for me to go to typing classes. So, at 15, I began work as a junior in the office of Hunt's Typewriter Services in St. Giles and then, about three years later, I began training as a medical secretary in the Pathology Department at the Radcliffe Infirmary. At about this time, Alan and I began going out together and six years later, when I was 23, we married. For about 18 months we lived with my mother-in-law but, early in 1967, we were able to move into our own home.

With the exception of the time when I was really ill with agoraphobia I have worked all my adult life. When we were first married, I was employed as a receptionist and switchboard operator with an insurance company but shortly afterwards I returned to work as a medical secretary and was then with various doctors at the Radcliffe Infirmary, Oxford.

2

The Panic Attacks Begin

I know exactly when the attacks began. It was in 1967 when I was still employed by the insurance company. Several of the girls at the office had read about a new diet which was currently all the rage, and we decided to try it. It was reputed to 'clear the system', and involved drinking a brand of pure lemon juice (PLJ) and restricting food intake to a very plain, low-calorie diet. After adhering to the PLJ part of the plan strictly for a week as required, I became tired of the limited range of food allowed and resumed normal eating. It was at this point that all my troubles began. The direct cause was not the PLJ diet but the fact that, after a break from what I eventually found to be 'forbidden' foodstuffs, I began to eat them again. It was only much later that I was to discover that the attacks were triggered by what I was eating.

It was my lunch hour and I was walking along Walton Street to my grandmother's house. After having been taken ill at my wedding, she never left her bed again and I usually visited her each lunchtime during the week because we enjoyed the other's company so much. We had always been very close. It was a clear sunny day, I remember, cold but nice and I was walking along quite happily. I had to cross the road to the long grey wall of Worcester College but while crossing, I had a strange feeling come over me and an urgent need simply to get to the other side. I was able to do so but as I reached the pavement I experienced the most dreadful sensation that I was about to loose consciousness. I stopped dead in my tracks. My vision became misty, my heart was thumping, my hands began to sweat, my whole body was trembling with fear. My legs had become so weak and unsteady that I found it difficult to stand. I was terrified by what was happening to me. It was impossible to understand and I seriously thought that I was about to die. All I wanted was for someone to help me. Desperately I tried to attract anyone's attention but I was completely unable to utter a single word. Finally, someone did pass by and I was somehow able to let them know that I was feeling ill and ask if they would get me a taxi. This they did from a nearby rank. I knew it would take only a short time for the taxi to arrive from Gloucester Green but I doubted that I would survive. But come it did and took me the final few hundred yards to my grandmother's house. It truly was such a short distance but I would have found it quite impossible to walk there even if my life had really depended on it.

When I reached the house, my mother was there and immediately she realised that I was having a panic attack since both she and my grandmother had experienced the same problem in the past. Indeed, two relatives had also had similar trouble but at the time I was in such a state that I was only concerned with what was happening to me then and there. Mother paid off the taxi and she and my grandmother both set about reassuring me over a cup of tea as I sat on the setee in the small front room.

After that attack I completely lost my confidence to go out alone and had to take six weeks sick leave from work. My father-in-law would take me to my grandmother's each day in his car and during the brief period I was there I would rest quietly on the setee, having first taken the tranquillisers that my doctor had prescribed for me.

Thus began years of torture to both my mind and body. I was unable to sit still even in my own home. Strangely, I was affected by the weather, especially by heavy rain, and if I felt more frightened than usual I would telephone a neighbour who would come and sit with me until I improved.

Shopping proved to be an absolute nightmare. I had to park the car as near as I possibly could to the shops, a very considerable problem in a city with such horrendous parking difficulties as Oxford's. On one occasion, I had to produce a letter from my G.P. to explained why it was necessary for me to park my car on a yellow line.

The problem affected practically every aspect of my life. Whenever I went in a supermarket I always had to be aware of the exits so that I could escape. In fact, I frequently had to abandon my trolley and its contents and run out of the store. I had to make an excuse if someone wanted to stop and talk with me. For many years my social life was, to all intents and purposes, non-existent.

When I was invited to a party or dance I took a double dose of Valium in order to get there and then I had to sit near an exit all the time. I found it quite impossible to force myself to the middle of the floor to dance and so would spend the evening watching the clock go round and praying for the function to end. All I wanted was the safety of my own home. My hairdresser had to visit me at home because I was incapable of sitting in a salon. After my sons were born I would start out to take them to the cinema but invariably would have to turn back before we got there. Constantly I was being told to pull myself together or that what I really needed was a good kick up the backside! But I just felt exhausted all the time and practically useless as a wife and mother.

My doctor was very good, but about all he could prescribe was Valium. I told him of the feelings of fright that I had had for such a long time and how they had become worse since my marriage. He did his best for me; he always came to see me whenever I asked but it was mainly a matter of giving me more pills. They must have been effective to some extent because I was able to resume work, but I was constantly on edge waiting for the next attack to begin.

3

More Attacks

Although, over the course of the years, I had suffered many attacks and all were frightening to different degrees, several stick in my mind.

When my grandmother died, my mother lived in the Walton Street house and at the end of my visits to her I used to take a taxi home because of the apprehension I felt when I travelled by public transport. Derek, my first child, was about 18 months old and we had been to see mother when I felt particularly ill in the taxi. As soon as we reached my house I bundled everything indoors, Derek, the pushchair, my bag, and ran as quickly as I could down the road to one of my neighbours. Luckily she was in and she tried to convince me that I was not on the verge of death. I knew better, of course, and finally persuaded her to call me a taxi to take me back to my mother.

I ran in with Derek, thrust him into mother's arms and told her that I was going over the road to the casualty department at the Radcliffe Infirmary. I had to get there before I died. Mother's arguments that I had been through all this many times before and yet I was still alive fell on deaf ears. This time was different, I knew it. All she could do was to stand there feeling genuinely sorry for me. She is an undemonstrative person who finds it difficult to show her true feelings. But I knew that Derek would be safe with her as I dashed across the road to the Infirmary. Walton Street is a busy main road and, on reflection, it is interesting to realise that, terrified as I was, I must have taken great care to avoid the traffic.

I knew exactly where the casualty department was and how to get to it because I had at one time worked on the floor above it. Along a little pathway, up lots of steps, through a door, then another set of doors and down a long corridor I ran as fast as my legs would carry me. I never stopped to consider how I could possibly have done that if, as I felt, I was about to die from a heart attack.

Breathlessly, I told the receptionist that I needed to see a doctor immediately. I was put on a couch and into a gown. A doctor arrived quite quickly and after a brief examination left me with a promise to return in a minute. I watched the second hand on the wall clock go round convinced that by the time a full minute had elapsed I would be dead.

When the doctor returned he was sympathetic.

'You're as strong as an ox,' he said after listening to my heart. 'You'll outlive me.'

Having thus cheered me up, he reassured me that there was nothing at all wrong with my heart but that the cause of such extreme anxiety had to be found. He left me with the advice that I should see my own doctor to find out what the real cause of my problem was.

But nothing really changed after that attack. Our second son, Clive, had been born when a group of us, Alan, me and our two boys, my mother-in-law, and two brothers-in-law, one with his wife and their two small girls and the other with his girl friend, spent a holiday at Portland Bill on the south coast. We had had a lovely fortnight and for our final meal before driving home we visited *The Lobster Pot.* I had just ordered my lunch when the usual feeling of impending death flooded over me. As I reached for my tranquillisers, Alan knew from the look on my face what was wrong and asked his brother Richard to fetch his car. On this occasion, however, I was able to compose myself somewhat and I just sat there sipping a Coca Cola as I took my Valium. In this way I was able to survive the long journey back to Oxford.

As soon as we got home I remember that the first thing I did was to put my head under the cold water tap.

'*Now* can we get a doctor?', I asked Alan.

Although, on the face of it, it might have seemed unnecessary, Alan knew better. He was like that. He always did what I asked, just going along with me. He had learned to cope with my panics, though the aches and pains and palpitations were another matter. The doctor who came was fairly new to the practice and so gave me a thorough examination. He found that my heart was fine and in answer to my query about the cause he said that he could find nothing at all physically wrong with me. At the same time, he did not believe that it was entirely in my mind.

'Have you thought about diet?', he asked.

That was something that had never been put to us directly before and we simply looked at him in amazement. Certainly it had been one of the many ideas we had been aware of but we had never previously followed it up. Now we did so and as a result I went to Basingstoke Hospital to see Dr. Richard Mackarness who had published a book on the subject, *Not All in the Mind.*

4

The Boys

My sons were my life. Since Derek was born, followed three years later by Clive, I had always tried to hide my feelings of panic from them. It was not easy, but I did not want them to grow up afraid. Like any other children, they were constantly wanting to go somewhere and I would frequently make preparations only to have to apologise and cancel everything at the very last minute.

They loved to go swimming and we would often pack everything into the car and set out for the pool in North Oxford, then turn back because I felt terrible. Sometimes, I would park in a side street and make them wait in the car while I went into a shop for a bottle of Coca Cola so that I could take my tranquilliser. Then we could carry on. Or I would call at my mother's and ask her to come with us because I was feeling unwell. On most of these occasions she did come.

The boys began their education at the local North Hinksey village school before we sent them to Josca's, a very good private school at Frilford Heath. I was determined that I would always support them by attending all their functions no matter how I was feeling, even if I had to force myself to do so. So, when the school's Christmas Carol service came round, I promised to go. It meant quite a long drive down dark and lonely country roads, but I got there. The service was held in the big school hall and it was packed with pupils and parents; there was standing room only. As I stood at the back, feeling quite certain that the tranquilliser I had taken had had no effect, I saw Alan's G.P, so I worked my way through to a position immediately in front of him. I felt safe with him there and I was able to stay for the whole service.

But not all outings were negotiated so successfully. In Oxford the St. Giles Fair is held annually each September and the boys looked forward to it every year. Personally, I dreaded its approach. Derek was almost ten, Clive was nearly seven, and I was feeling far from well when the time for the fair came round. Knowing how much they had been looking forward to it and not wanting to disappoint them, I knew that we had to go. I drove there, parked the car and we walked a little way into the fair, which by this time was going full blast. It is a huge fair, taking up the whole of St. Giles in the centre of Oxford. Every ride imaginable is there; the Big Wheel, space rides, the Wall of Death, bumper cars, roundabouts, and much more. Even at 11.30 in the morning the noise was overpowering, and we had planned to spend the whole day there!

We got only as far as the Wimpey Bar on the edge of the fair when I had to tell the boys that we would have to go back home. Clive threw a tantrum and refused to leave. I became upset and felt even more unwell and then Derek, too, began protesting and refusing to go home with me. The last thing I wanted was for them to see me having a major attack in the street, but I also knew that if I stayed I would pass out with fear. As I saw it, my only course was to start back on my own. Fortunately, crying their eyes out, the boys followed me back to the car. All the way home the crying continued, which made me feel even worse, and the accusations flew thick and fast.

'You've let us down again! We always start off somewhere and end up going home before we've had any fun.'

Unfortunately, I had no answer to that.

5

Back to Work

When my sons had both started school, my mother suggested to me that I might like to get myself a little job. She thought it might take my mind off the panic attacks but I was far from sure that it would. It was shortly afterwards, that I happened to see an advertisement for a position as part time medical secretary at the Radcliffe Infirmary working with Dr. Burke, a consultant endocrinologist. I applied for the job and was granted an interview.

When the time came, I asked mother to come along with me for moral support. Because I had worked at the Radcliffe before, I knew where Dr. Burke's office was and mother and I walked together down the long corridor, she with her hand in the small of my back gently propelling me in the right direction. She was taking no chances that I would turn tail and run, though halfway along the corridor I did stop and say that I felt unable to go any further. She insisted, however, and with a little extra pressure from her hand we made it the rest of the way.

She waited as I went upstairs to see Dr. Burke and the personnel officer. All the usual questions were asked and answered until finally Dr. Burke, a really charming man, asked me as he sat gently tapping his pipe if I felt there was anything else I would like to tell them. How could I say that this grown, married woman sitting before them applying for a responsible job had her mother downstairs waiting to take her home? I could see the amusing side of it but I told them quite simply that I suffered from panic attacks and that I felt they ought to be aware of that, even though it might cost me any chance of being appointed. Dr. Burke, being a physcian, must have realised the implications of that information but he thought for a moment or two and the said they would let me know.

I went home thinking that was the end of the matter and I had just made myself a cup of tea when the telephone rang. It was Dr. Burke who told me that they would like to offer me the job. Although it was, as advertised, a part time appointment, eventually I worked in the office on a full time basis.

I would frequently feel panic rising as I made my way to work in my car and would want to turn round and go home, but on those occasions I would hear my grandmother saying, 'If at first you don't succeed . . .' My heart would be pounding but I would refuse to give in. When I could, I would take another Valium and get back into the stream of traffic and carry on to the hospital. I always parked my car under the window of Dr. Burke's office and I would make my way from the security of the car to the security of the office as quickly as possible.

Dr. Burke did not always realise what a struggle it had been for me to get to the office. I tried all the time to follow my grandmother's advice to remain cheerful and take care of my appearance. There is a great tendency when you feel permanently unwell to let personal standards slip and I was determined that was not going to happen to me. At least Dr. Burke seemed satisified.

'Deanna,' he would say, 'you're like a ray of sunshine coming into the office each morning.'

6

The Medical Establishment

Not infrequently I was literally afraid to go to sleep at night in case I did not wake up again. Sleepless nights were a real problem. They got in the way of both my work and Alan's. When I felt frightened, Alan would try to calm me, to settle me down and reassure me that I would be fine in the morning. When I told him that my heart was racing so much that I feared it would stop, he reminded me how many times I had been told by doctors just how strong it was. But when I wanted to go downstairs in the middle of the night he was not always too pleased at having his sleep disturbed! Sometimes, however, he would get up with me; at other times I would just creep out of bed and go down alone.

Of course I did everything I could think of to discover what was making me feel so unwell. At one point I thought that it might be a hormonal or hereditary problem since both my mother and my grandmother had had the same trouble. What I really needed and longed for more than anything else in the world was to find a doctor who could tell me that he knew there was something wrong with me, that he knew exactly what it was, and that he could cure it.

My G.P. referred me to a specialist. I had to go to see him as a private patient because I would have suffered a panic attack waiting in a long queue of National Health Service patients. This doctor, a consultant physician at Oxford and highly regarded by the medical profession, still sits on a number of boards. I was at my lowest ebb as he examined me and then told me he could find nothing wrong. I asked him if I could make another appointment for a year's time to which his reply was,

'No, you can't see me again. You are simply a neurotic woman. I'll write to your G.P. and explain.'

He did send a letter to my G.P. suggesting that I should be prescribed a drug which I later discovered may cause Parkinson's disease if taken in large quantities.

Several doctors diagnosed my fears as agoraphobia despite the fact that the attacks were just as likely to happen at home as out of doors. Others told me that I was imagining the whole thing. I remember being referred to a physician, who was later knighted, at the John Radcliffe. It was during the school holidays so that my two sons and a friend's child that I was looking after were with me. Although I felt dreadful on that particular day, we took a taxi to the hospital where I was eventually shown into his very imposing consulting room. I asked if he could do something to help me immediately as I was having an acute attack at that very minute and I had to get the three boys home as quickly as possible. After a quick examination he said,

'Well, there's nothing wrong with you but what I will do, my dear, is refer you to one of my friends.'

Whenever they say that you know that they are talking about a psychiatrist.

I did see 'one of his friends' at the Warneford Hospital in Oxford. His name was Dr. Nutt! A friend had dropped me off there and I was feeling particularly anxious because I was alone. As I was sitting in his waitingroom, I began to doodle on a piece of paper and wrote 'What am I doing in a place like this? I know this hospital hasn't got the answer.' I had the piece of paper in my hand as I went in to see the doctor. Immediately, he asked if he could see what I had been writing and I handed the paper over, thinking that it would be useful for him to know how I felt. On the basis of what I had written, he diagnosed me as having 'a histrionic personality given to oscillating between physical and psychological ailments'. He wanted me to try group therapy but I was not prepared to agree to that. Deep down I knew that whatever was wrong with me the cause was physical not psychological.

I reached the stage where I began to think that I did not count for very much. Now, I feel sufficiently well informed to discuss the subject with doctor. Not only were so many of them so wrong in their diagnosis and treatment of me, but I have worked with enough of them to know their weaknesses as well as their strengths. I will speak out to any member of the medical profession and tell them that they do not always have the answers. And that includes the practitioners of alternative medicine too. In my time, I have tried acupuncture, deep breathing, yoga, meditation, even hypnosis but although my general health was improved to a certain degree by some of these, none had any really significant influence on my main problem, the panic attacks. A friend even took me to a healing service at which I knelt at the altar with a priest. Nothing and no one could help me.

7

Dr. Ritchie and the Diet

The first hint of a possible connection between diet and my illness had come many years earlier, after our holiday at Portland Bill, from one of the doctors at the practice. He asked if I would mind being referred to a doctor who had written a book on allergy and diet. I would have to see him as a private patient but, after many attempts to find a cure, I was prepared to go to any lengths. So, with Alan's agreement to pay the fee, we made the arrangements.

A friend drove me to Basingstoke Hospital where I saw Dr. Richard Mackarness, the author of *Not All in the Mind*. He put me on what he called his 'Stone Age Diet', details of which are given in his book. It was a tough regime and I followed it to the letter. However, I felt no better afterwards. So I discontinued the diet and in the following years I assumed that such treatment could not help me.

In 1984 I began to suffer from severe stomach pains and a distended abdomen. A doctor at the John Radcliffe Hospital at Oxford suspected a cancerous growth, but fortunately his diagnosis proved to be incorrect. It was at that stage that a friend suggested to me that I might like to go to see Dr. Ritchie, a gastroenterologist, in case he could help. When I kept my appointment with him I was suffering from terrible abdominal pains, and diets and such like treatments were the last things on my mind.

I had become accustomed by this time to paying for private consultations and going to see impressive-looking physcians in their elegant offices with receptionists and nurses in attendance. So I was more than surprised when Dr. Ritchie himself opened the door to his Banbury Road premises and welcomed me in. He was a short, unassuming, greyish man with a very pleasant manner and, unlike most of the other private consultants I had seen, he was not wearing the usual pin-striped suit. From that first meeting his straightforwardness put me at ease, especially so on that first visit when I was troubled with chronic indigestion. I kept belching, apologising, and immediately belching again!

'No need to be embarrassed,' he said, 'I know exactly how you feel. Now, tell me all about yourself.'

'You mean about my tummy?'

'Yes, but tell me also about the panics and the palpitations.'

He had learned of these from my G.P.'s letter.

'Oh, and are you going to tell me that I'm neurotic, just like all the others have done?', I said.

'No, no you're not neurotic,' he said quietly, 'It's nothing to do with that.'

I remember his soft voice and how relaxed I had become as I sat there. I told him how other members of my family had also suffered from panic attacks, palpitations and depressions and asked him if such a condition could be hereditary.

'Yes, most definitely,' he answered and went on to ask me more questions.

It seemed that I had been there only a very short time when he said,

'I'm going to give you a diet and I would like you to follow it strictly for two weeks. Then come to see me again to tell me how you are.'

I was still under the impression that this was all connected with my abdominal pains. After all, he *was* a gastroenterologist. His parting words were,

'Even if you feel tempted, don't break the diet at all. Stick exactly to what I've told you.'

The diet sheets he had handed me had been devised by Dr. Hunter of Addenbrookes Hospital, Cambridge.

I felt more relaxed on the journey home. I stopped at a health food shop and bought soya milk and herb teas and several other items that were included in the diet. I had seen Dr. Ritchie on a Wednesday and I was to begin the diet the next day, Thursday. I got up that morning feeling my usual self, that is to say not at all well, but I began the diet as planned. After doing all my usual jobs around the house I had to go out in the car. The open air still made me apprehensive, in fact it was a normal day in every respect. Similarly the next day. I stuck to the diet but felt no differently except that, in the afternoon, I had a real throbbing headache, far worse than my usual headaches. By the time Alan came home from work I had to lie down because the pain was so great. Dr. Ritchie had warned me that if I experienced any aches or pains, under no circumstances was I to take anything to relieve them as this would interfere with the diet. So I heeded his advice and went to bed early, hoping that the headache was nothing serious.

I slept reasonably well. Next morning, the headache had gone when I got up and went into the kitchen to make myself a cup of herbal tea. But something I could not quite put my finger on was different about the daily routine. Certainly the abdominal pains had gone, but that was not too surprising. The diet would have taken care of them, wouldn't it? And then it struck me. I felt *relaxed and well,* at peace with the world. I wanted to believe it but it was so uncanny that I found it almost impossible to do so. I carried on making the herbal tea and preparing breakfast for Alan and the boys and the feeling of disbelief continued. It was almost too good to be true so, not wanting to raise any false hopes for anyone, and especially for not me, I packed all the family off for the day as I usually did without saying a word about how I was feeling.

Even after I had been alone for a while I still felt the same, so much so that I had the urge to walk, yes walk, to the shops instead of taking the car. It was something I had not even contemplated for so long that just thinking about it was like a minor miracle. The shops were only about half a mile away down the hill, perhaps a 15 minute walk, but it had been three years since I had attempted to make that apparently simple journey on foot.

But this time I made it and, what is perhaps more surprising, enjoyed the experience. All the time I was expecting that the panic would begin and was surprised when it failed to do so. I remember the simple thigs so vividly, like looking into people's gardens, and seeing new paint on someone's gate, all the time thinking how strange, how unbelievable it was to be feeling so well.

When I reached the supermarket I would normally have made certain that I could, if I needed to, make a rapid exit. On this occasion it barely entered my head. I was not at all anxious and I thoroughly enjoyed being able to do my shopping at leisure. I was even able to stand in the queue at the checkout without any fear at all and then walk back home up the hill just as anyone else would expect to do. I felt marvellous. The change in me was sufficient for one neighbour to remark how strange it was to see Dee walking to the shops, something she had not seen for such a long time!

That, then, was the beginning of my improvement although I did not entirely appreciate it at the time. I obviously had some doubts that it was all going to last. Each day I felt a little better and, although I was still taking the Valium tablets I had been prescribed for years, I began to sense that I was no longer dependant on them. Not surprisingly, I stuck strictly to the diet Dr. Ritchie had given me and went back to see him at the time we had arranged.

'Well, you're not going to believe this but I've never felt better in my life. In fact, I want to know if I can start coming off the Valium.'

I could hardly wait to get into the room before I began reporting my progress to Dr. Ritchie.

'Why do you think I'm not going to believe it?'

'Because I feel so well.'

He half smiled, I remember, as he said that he was not at all surprised.

'But I thought I was seeing you just for my abdominal problems.'

'Oh no. As soon as you walked through that door and heard you speak with that nasal tone I knew that you had a food intolerance. Knowing about your chronic indigestion, the nasal tone was very important. The two together indicate food intolerance. In nine cases out of ten, panic attacks together with indigestion and nasal problems can mean that it's a diet-related illness. So I was not at all surprised by your improvement. As for the Valium, you can slowly reduce the dose until you eliminate it altogether.'

It was still some time ahead, but I was finally able to consider myself free of my dependence on Valium after 15 years and I suffered virtually no withdrawal symptoms.

It was imperative that the diet was followed to the letter for those first two weeks. After that, the most difficult task was to discover what I could and could not eat.

'When you leave here,' Dr. Ritchie told me, 'I want you to introduce one item at a time from this list of forbidden foods.'

He gave me instructions on how to do this. When I introduced milk, for example, I had to drink a glass in the morning and if I showed no reaction by teatime, I had to drink another glass then. If, when I woke the next morning, I felt at all unwell, then from that time onwards milk would be barred from my diet. I had to wait for three days for the milk to clear my system before I could test the next item on the list.

Wheat took the longest time to test with 24 hours to produce an adverse reaction. I had to eat two wheat rolls for breakfast and another two at night then look for a reaction the following day. It came.

As Dr. Ritchie said, 'Apart from an occasional sandwich, I'm afraid you're off that for the rest of your life.'

Corn had a dramatic effect and that also includes glucose syrup, which is derived from corn. I shudder when I recall that I used to eat corn flakes every day of my life and I also added sugar and poured on milk! I have the vivid recollection of my mother adding massive amounts of sugar from the sugar basin and eating lots of bread, usually white. We always ate bread. And I used to take my Valium with Coca Cola, just about the worst thing I could possibly have done! All the items were on the list and from that time on I did not taste them for years although I do now indulge myself very infrequently with very small amounts.

Each day for four months I kept a detailed diary in which I recorded the time I got up, what I ate, what I drank, and how I felt. I saw Dr. Ritchie every week during those four months. At our meetings we religiously went through my diary, gradually introducing different foodstuffs and noting whether they had any effect on me. It took patience, it was extremely time-consuming, and sometimes very complicated. But I cared nothing about that because the other side of the coin was that it was working. I was getting better; I was beginning to live again!

8

Disappointing Dates

For the first time in years I was not having to rely on Valium. I had been on my strict diet for two years and was feeling fine but, at the same time, I was beginning to feel bored constantly eating the same bland food. I felt in urgent need of a little variety as I toured the local shops. Seeing a box of dates at the greengrocers I knew that they would provide me with the treat I was looking for but caution had become second nature by this time and I asked the greengrocer, whom I knew quite well, whether the date contained any additives.

'Not as far as I know.' he said, 'They're just what it says on the box, plain dates.'

Having been reassured, I bought a box and took it home with the intention of sharing the dates with my mother-in-law when she came to tea on Sunday. It may seem greedy, but we ate the whole box between us. To be honest, she ate a couple and I had the rest! But I enjoyed them. They had been tasty and filling, and I promised myself that I would get another box whenever I felt the need to have a treat again.

The following morning, after Alan had gone to work, I remember going to the bathroom and being aware of the onset of one of those feelings I had not experienced for two years. The diet, I thought, had finally let me down. I really felt too frightened to go downstairs but forced myself to do so and I sat on the bottom stair to telephone Dr. Ritchie. Luckily he was in his office and I quickly told him how ill I was feeling and that the diet was not working any more.

'But that's not possible, Mrs. Peedell. We've established beyond doubt that the diet works. Now just calm down and tell me exactly what you've eaten, especially anything that's on the forbidden list.'

Although I told him that I had not strayed from the diet, he made me go through every single thing that I had eaten or drunk. When I got as far as the dates he interrupted me.

'Was the brand name Eat Me?'

'Yes, but dates are not on the forbidden list.'

'No,' he said, 'but corn syrup is.'

'But the greengrocer told me that there were no additives.'

'Well there are no additives named on the box, but these dates are dipped in corn syrup. That's what makes them so sweet. If you'd eaten just a single date you might have got away with it but you've been off corn for years so it's not surprising that the massive dose you gave yourself brought on such a panic.'

I was tremendously impressed by Dr. Ritchie's confidence. He *knew* the diet was effective. It had just been a matter of finding the substance that had triggered the attack and in this case it had not taken him long.

I am pleased to say that the importers have now added the information about the syrup to the label on the box, but it must be remembered that all sweets contain glucose syrup as do lots of baby foods, Ribena, etc. The list is endless.

It is encouraging to see that, over the last few years, so much more has been discovered about the connection between allergies and food additives and that the wrappings of a great many more products, even of the plainest packet of biscuits, have all the ingredients listed.

9

St. Giles Fair Revisited

The discovery of the way diet could control my panic attacks and so have such a profound affect on my life is typified by one outing I had with the boys. Derek was about fourteen and Clive about eleven. It was some four years after that dreadful visit to St. Giles Fair to which I referred earlier. The contrast between the two occasions could not have been greater. Whereas we were not able even to start enjoying the attractions that first time, now we explored the whole length of the fair and tried everything. I felt so well and was determined to show the boys that Mum knew how to enjoy herself like the best of them. I had no feelings of panic at all and to see their faces as they sampled ride after ride, well . . .

That visit to the fair was the pinnacle of the whole wonderful process. I had quite literally been reborn. I walked for miles and enjoyed the scenery, I spent hours in town browsing through the shops, I visited all the large food stores and strolled to the hair salon alone or with a friend. For the first time in ages I thrilled to be able to travel by bus!

Not only were Alan and my mother happy for me, they also enjoyed a huge benefit themselves from my being able to lead a normal life. My mother's own health improved when she followed my example and her panics ceased after she gave up eating sugar and eggs.

My younger son, Clive, has now qualified as a doctor and hopes to be able to make a study of diet later in his career. My other son, Derek, has so far experienced no serious health problems and is pursuing a career in banking. Even during the worst of my nightmare years I must have been doing something right for them. Alan and I made sure that their education was unaffected and they both went to Magdalen College School after leaving Josca's. They could so easily have taken advantage of my problems and run riot, or dropped out, or got themselves into all manner of bother, and who could have blamed them? Despite the fact that I felt I had let them down so badly during their formative years, I have a sense of pride that they are now doing so well and I thank them.

My grandmother was a very important person in my life. It was she who gave me the will to persevere and when things were difficult I could hear her constantly urging me on,

'If you want anything in life you have to work for it. Remember, it doesn't come to you; you've got to go to it.'

Most importantly, she would tell me never to give up. There were so very many occasions when I felt that there was nothing I would like to do more than just give up, but then I would hear her voice just as clearly as if she was standing next to me,

'You just carry on girl . . .'

10

The Exclusion Diet

It cannot be repeated too frequently nor stated too strongly that you should never, under any circumstances, embark on an exclusion diet without first consulting a doctor or a dietician who will give you full instructions on how to proceed.

The next few pages contain details of the classes of food that should be excluded entirely from your diet and those which are permitted. A regime using only the permitted foods is normally continued for two weeks and from the day you begin it you must keep a detailed record of everything you eat and drink as well as any medication you take. Examples of my own records during the time I was undergoing this period of testing are given in the Appendix. It is most important that you also record at the same time exactly how you are feeling.

After the two weeks, you will be instructed to add one of the previously forbidden foods to your diet. For example, I have described in section 7 how it was demonstrated that I was intolerant to both milk and wheat and it is necessary to repeat this process for each food with a period of three days on the exclusion diet between the end of testing one food and the beginning of testing the next. There is, unfortunately, no short cut.

Inevitably, the whole process of establishing exactly what you may safely include in your diet and what you must rigorously avoid is a long one possibly fraught with many disappointments. You are almost certain to discover that you react to some of your favourite foods. But if you want to improve your health they must go; there is no alternative.

Excluded foods

It is essential that **every trace** of the following items of food should be removed from your diet for two weeks. Listed on this page are the broad classes of foods to be excluded but it should be noted that it is sometimes possible that the contents of a package will not be described using exactly these terms. Alternative names are therefore listed on the following page. If you come across something about which you are uncertain, always check whether it is allowed before eating it.

Cereals

Wheat
Corn
Oats
Rye
Barley

Dairy

Milk
Cheese
Butter
Yoghurt

Meats and Fish

Bacon
Cooked meats
Smoked meats
  and fish
Beef

Fruits

Citrus fruits

Vegetables

Onions
Potato
Cabbage
Sprouts
Peas

Miscellaneous

Coffee
Eggs
Tea
Chocolate
Nuts
Additives
Yeast/sugar

Among the alternative names for excluded foods are

Wheat: Flour, semolina, pasta, bran, wheat-germ (natural Vitamin E), rusk, crouton, breadcrumbs.

Corn: (maize) i.e. sweet corn, cornflour, maize semolina, corn oil (Mazola), maize-germ oil, corn syrup, edible starch, glucose, dextrose, dextrins, gin, vodka, liqueurs. Present as filler in most medicinal tablets and pills (test with iodine: starch produces a blue colour with a solution of iodine).

Barley: includes malt, e.g. beer, whisky, vinegar.

Milk: includes fresh, dried, skimmed, long-life, condensed, etc. Whey (in soft margarines). All dairy and goat milk products.

Beef: includes dripping, stock cubes, extracts, veal, gelatin.

Citrus: includes oranges, lemons, limes, grapefruit, etc. and their juices, marmalades.

Coffee: includes instant, decaffeinated, essence.

Tea: Indian, China, Earl Grey.

Nuts: all kinds, e.g. almonds, hazels, brazils, peanuts, etc. and all nut products.

Additives: includes colours, synthetic flavours and flavour enhancers, antioxidants, preservatives, etc.
Record the E number of any additives eaten with goods in the diary.

Yeast: Marmite, Vit B tablets.

Permitted foods

You may eat any of the following unless you know that they upset you.

Cereals	Meats and Fish	Fruits
Rice	Pork	Apples
Millet	Chicken	Rhubarb
Sago	(not frozen)	Banana
Tapioca	Lamb	Strawberry
Buckwheat	Turkey	Pineapple
Gram flour	White fish	Pear
Soya flour	Shell fish	Grapes
		Melon
		Avocado
		Raspberry

Vegtables		Miscellaneous
Carrots	Soya bean	Wine
Lettuce	Marrow	Tap water
Leeks	Broccoli	Saccharine
Spinach	Beetroot	Honey
Mushroom	Peppers	
Parsnips	Tomato	
Cauliflower	Celery	
Green beans	Cucumber	
Turnip		

Try to vary your daily choice of foods. For example:

Day 1: Meat, 1–2 fruits, 2–3 vegetables at main meals.
Day 2: Chicken, different fruits, different vegetables.
Day 3: Fish, etc.

Among the alternative names for the permitted foods are

Rice:	Preferably brown rice, including rice products, e.g. rice, flour, 'rice cakes'.
Other grains and flours:	Sago, tapioca, millet, buckwheat, gram flour, soya flour.
Milk:	Use soya milk (liquid form, not dried and not containing glucose syrup).
Margarine:	Use Tomor or Granose margarine.
Cooking oil:	Use 'vegetable', sunflower, safflower or olive oil.
Vinegar:	Use cider vinegar or wine vinegar.
Hot drinks:	Try dandelion coffee or perhaps herb teas (tissances), e.g. camomile, rose hip, peppermint, etc.
Dietary bulk:	Soya bran.

If you are unable to find any of the listed items in your local supermarket, try any good health food store. They are invaluable sources for the foods you will require.

An extremely useful book is *The Allergy Diet,* written by Workman, Hunter and Alun Jones, published in paperback by Optima and priced at £5.00.

My diet has become a way of life to me over the years and I have found it easy to feed a hungry husband and two strapping sons without them going hungry or me 'poisoning' my system. In the following pages I give recipes which are just a sample of the many delicious and nutritious dishes I have discovered and/or adapted. They are quick and easy to prepare and economical. If you want to impress, I have found that the avocado and prawn dish never fails to do just that.

Breakfast Mixture

millet flakes
sunflower seeds
fructose
dried apricots
raisins

Eat the mixture with soya milk, pure honey and stewed fruit.

Kedgeree

½ cup brown rice
Small fillet of cod or other fleshy white fish
2 oz./50 g cooked chick peas
1 tomato

Dot the fish with Granose margarine, sprinkle with herbs and grill until tender.
Cook the rice and skin and flake the fish. Melt a dessertspoonful of oil or Granose margarine in a frying pan, mix in the fish and rice and heat through. Add the peas.
Serve with sliced tomato on top and chopped parsley.

Vegetable Soup

About 2 lbs. of mixed fresh vegetables, e.g. carrots, leeks, parsnips, cauliflower, peas, skinned tomatoes
2 soya stock cubes
½ pint soya milk
Granose margarine
1 heaped teaspoon of mixed herbs
salt and pepper to taste

Roughly chop up all the vegetables. Melt about one desertspoonful of Granose margarine in a large saucepan and sauté the vegetables for a few minutes.

Add enough boiling water to just cover the vegetables and crumble in the stock cubes. Add the herbs, salt and pepper, and stir. Cover the pan and simmer on a low heat until the vegetables are soft. Add the soya milk and stir.

Either liquidise the soup in an electric blender or purée it through a sieve. Check the seasoning before serving.

This soup is suitable for freezing.

Lentil and Bean Soup

6 oz./170 g red lentils
1 small can of broad beans, washed and drained
1 small can of red kidney beans, washed and drained
1 stick of celery and/or 1 leek
5 fl. oz. soya milk
1 teaspoon herbs
black pepper and salt

Soak the lentils overnight. Place them in a saucepan with ½ pint of water and add the coarsely chopped celery and/or leek, the herbs, and salt and pepper. Bring to the boil then reduce the heat and simmer for 10 minutes.

Add the beans and soya milk and cook for a further 10 minutes. Blend in an electric blender for a few seconds or, alternatively, mash the beans well with a fork.

Serve sprinkled with a little chopped parsley.

Stuffed Peppers

1 pepper, de-seeded
1 small cup brown rice
4 oz./100 g lean pork, chopped into small cubes
1 oz./25 g raisins, washed
1 oz./25 g cooked or tinned red kidney beans
1 soya stock cube
½ teaspoon mixed herbs
paprika
salt and black pepper
oil

Pre-heat the oven to 170° C/350° F/Gas 4.

Put the pepper in a saucepan and cover with water. Bring it to the boil and then simmer for 5 minutes. Remove from the heat and drain. Cook the brown rice in water to which a soya stock cube has been added.

Meanwhile, heat about a tablespoon of oil in a frying pan and when hot, sauté the pork and herbs in it. Sprinkle the pork generously with paprika while it is cooking. When it is tender remove from the heat and add the beans and raisins. Mix all this with the cooked rice and use the mixture to stuff the pepper firmly.

Place the stuffed pepper in a small ovenproof dish and surround it with any remaining rice mixture. Cover the dish with foil and bake for 45–60 minutes.

Serve with a tomato salad or a spicy tomato sauce.

Sweet and Sour Pork with Bean Sprouts and Rice

1 small cup brown rice
4 oz./100 g lean pork cut into very thin 1 inch pieces
2 oz./50 g pineapple, cut into small pieces
1 green pepper, thinly sliced
1 carrot, thinly sliced
8 oz./200 g fresh beansprouts
1 tomato
soya sauce
1 dessertspoon ground ginger
½ teaspoon chilli powder (optional)
oil for frying

Put the rice on to cook and when it is about 10 minutes from being ready heat a tablespoon of oil in a wok or frying pan. When the oil is very hot, add the pork and fry, stirring quickly all the time so that it does not burn. As soon as the meat is well browned, reduce the heat and add the carrot and pepper. Sprinkle in the ginger, chilli powder (if used), black pepper and a few liberal shakes of soya sauce. Stir fry for 1 minute, then add the pineapple and bean sprouts and some more soya sauce. After a further minute add the chopped tomato. The mixture should now be moist and juicy and the vegetables cooked but still crunchy. Add some more soya sauce to taste for final flavouring and place on top of the cooked rice on a plate.

Avocado and Prawns with Yoghurt

avocado pear
2 oz./50 g fresh or thawed frozen prawns
2 tablespoons sheep's yoghurt
¼ teaspoon each of paprika, chilli powder and black pepper

Halve the avocado and remove the stone. Place the two halves on a dish and fill the centres with prawns.

Mix the spices into the sheep's yoghurt and top the prawns with it. Finish with a sprinkling of chopped herbs.

Chicken with Apricots

1 breast of chicken with skin and any fat removed
1 small tin of apricots in unsweetened juice
1 soya stock cube

Place the chicken in a small casserole or ovenproof dish. Empty the tin of apricots over it and squash the apricots down with a fork. Add a little water. Crumble the stock cube into the liquid and cover the dish with foil. Bake for half an hour in a pre-heated oven at 180° C/350° F/Gas 4 then stir the juice and cook uncovered for a further half hour.

Tuna Casserole

1 7 oz./175 g can of tuna, drained
About 6 oz./150 g cooked peas
1 small can red kidney beans, drained and washed
1½ tablespoons brown rice flour
½ teaspoon mixed herbs
1½ oz./37 g Granose margarine
8 fl oz./250 ml soya milk
sunflower seeds

Melt the Granose margarine in a saucepan, stir in the flour and mix until smooth. Gradually add the milk and whisk gently with a balloon whisk until the mixture boils and thickens.

Remove the pan from the heat and add the herbs, tuna, peas and beans. Season with salt and pepper and mix well. Pour into a small casserole dish and sprinkle with a layer of sunflower or sesame seeds or both.

Place the casserole in an oven preheated to 180° C/350° F/Gas 4 and bake for about 20 minutes.

Mixed Bean Salad

1 small can butter beans
1 small can red kidney beans
1 small can chick peas
tinned or cooked frozen or fresh broad beans
¼ clove of garlic (optional)
sheep's milk yoghurt
unsweetened apple juice
Oregano, chives and mint

Drain the tinned beans and wash them. Combine all the beans in a bowl and sprinkle them generously with the oregano and chives, fresh if possible.

Mix 2 tablespoons of sheep's yoghurt with 1 teaspoon of apple juice. If you are using garlic, chop it finely and add it to the sheep's yoghurt. Trickle the sheep's yoghurt over the beans and then sprinkle with chopped mint and black pepper.

Spicy Tomato Sauce
(to accompany buckwheat spaghetti)

1 large tin tomatoes
2 tablespoons tomato purée
1 teaspoon pure honey
2 or 3 courgettes if in season
1 heaped teaspoon mixed oregano, thyme and basil
black pepper
salt to taste

Roughly chop the tinned tomatoes and place in a pan with the tomato purée. If you are using courgettes, slice them thinly crosswise and add them with the pure honey, herbs, salt and a generous amount of black pepper. Mix well and cover the pan. Simmer slowly until the sauce is thick and the courgettes soft.

Serve on cooked buckwheat spaghetti with grated or crumbled goat's cheese on top.

The sauce can also accompany roasted or grilled meat and can be stored in a fridge for several days or frozen.

Harvest Pie

Pastry case
4 oz./100 g chickpea (gram) flour
2 oz./50 g soya flour
3 oz./75 g Granose margarine
cold water

Sieve the dry ingredients into a bowl and rub in the Granose margarine. Gradually stir in the cold water and press together into a stiff dough. Roll out on a floured surface and line an 8 inch flan tin with it.

Put this aside in the fridge until the filling is ready.

Filling
14 oz./350 g unsweetened apple puree
6 oz./150 g washed chopped dates (fresh dates only)
3 oz./75 g washed raisins
3 oz./75 g washed and chopped dried figs
3 oz./75 g washed and chopped dried apricots
2 or 3 tablespoons pure honey
4 oz./100 g chopped sunflower seeds or millet flakes

Slowly simmer the apple puree, dried fruit and honey in an uncovered saucepan for about 15 minutes, stirring often. The mixture should then be very thick. Remove from the heat, cool, pour into the pastry case and top with the sunflower seed mixture. Bake for about 1 hour at 190° C/375° F/Gas 5 or until the pastry is cooked and the top lightly browned. Serve hot or cold, accompanied by sheep's yoghurt, ice cream, or a contrasting fruit purée such as strawberry, raspberry or blackcurrant.

Rhubarb Crumble

1 lb. rhubarb
3 tablespoons pure honey
1 teaspoon ground ginger
4 oz./100 g soya flour
4 oz./100 g rice flour
1½ tablespoons fructose
4 oz./100 g Granose margarine
2 oz./50 g millet flakes

Trim the rhubarb and cut into ½ inch pieces. Place in a casserole dish, trail the pure honey over and sprinkle with ground ginger.

In a bowl, combine the flours and rub in the Granose margarine until a breadcrumb consistency is reached. Add the fructose and millet flakes and mix in well. Sprinkle this over the rhubarb and press it down. Bake in a preheated oven at 180° C/350° F/Gas 4 for about 45 minutes.

Baked Banana

2 bananas, halved lengthways
1 tablespoon pure honey
2 tablespoons unsweetened pineapple juice
½ teaspoon cinnamon

Place the bananas in a shallow greased dish and spoon the pure honey and pineapple juice over them. Bake for 20 minutes in a preheated oven at 150° C/300° F/Gas 3. Serve alone or with sheep's yoghurt or fruit purée.

Mixed Fruit Fool

2 oz./50 g blackcurrants
2 oz./50 g raspberries
2 oz./50 g strawberries
1½ tablespoons fructose or 3 tablespoons pure honey
1 carton sheep's yoghurt

Top and tail the blackcurrants and place all the fruit in a pan with the sweetener. Heat very slowly. Allow to cook for a few minutes then either place in a blender and liquidise or mash to a pulp. Mix with the sheep's yoghurt and test for sweetness. Serve cold.

This dish can be made with other soft fruits such as rhubarb, apricots, and gooseberries.

Buckwheat and Rice Fritters

1 heaped tablespoon buckwheat flour
1 heaped tablespoon rice flour
pinch of salt
water

Sift the flours into a bowl and add the salt. Make a well in the centre and gradually add the water, stirring constantly, until a batter is formed. Use a balloon whisk for beating if the batter becomes lumpy.

Pour sufficient oil into a heavy frying pan to coat the base, heat and drop in enough of the batter to form a thin layer in the pan. Cook as for pancakes until crisp.

The fritters can be kept warm in a low oven. Serve hot.

Carob Flapjacks

4 oz./400 g Granose margarine
2 tablespoons pure honey
1 tablespoon carob powder
6 oz./150 g millet flakes

Pre-heat the oven to 180° C/350° F/Gas 4.

Melt the Granose margarine and pure honey in a saucepan. Stir in the carob powder and millet flakes and mix well. Press into a greased or non-stick 7 inch square or 7 inch diameter tin and bake for 15–20 minutes. When cool mark into squares.

Hot Chick Pea Bread

6 oz./150 g chick pea (gram) flour
2 teaspoons salt
1 teaspoon black pepper
5 fl. oz. sheep's milk yoghurt
2 oz./50 g Granose margarine

Sift the flour, salt and pepper into a bowl and gradually add the sheep's yoghurt to form a fairly stiff dough, adding a little water if necessary. Knead the dough until it is smooth then cover it and leave to stand for an hour.

Break off pieces of dough about 2½ inches/6 cm in diameter and roll them out into circles about $1/8$ inch thick. Melt the Granose margarine and brush it over the circles. Fold the circles up and roll them out again. Repeat the process twice more, finally rolling them out into circles of ¼ inch/½ cm thickness.

Dry fry the circles in a hot frying pan until golden brown on both sides and serve hot.

Brown Rice Crackers

3 oz./75 g brown rice flour
2½ oz./65 g millet flour
1 tablespoon soya flour
1 teaspoon cream of tartar
½ teaspoon bicarbonate of soda
½ teaspoon salt
1 oz. Granose, Tomor or similar margarine
3–4 tablespoons water

Place all the dry ingredients in a bowl and rub in the margarine. Gradually add cold water to make a ball of pastry-like consistency. This dough is difficult to handle, so roll out between two sheets of floured greaseproof paper to a thickness of $1/8$ inch. Remove the top sheet and cut the dough into approximately 2 inch squares.

Using a slice, transfer the squares to a greased baking sheet and bake for 5–7 minutes in a preheated oven at 200° C/400° F/Gas 6 until crisp. Remove from the baking sheet when cool.

Salad Dressing

Combine 1 dessertspoon of unsweetened apple juice with 1½ dessertspoons of oil. Add black pepper and a few pinches of herbs such as oregano, mint, and thyme, fresh if possible.

Fruit Purées

Most fruits can be made into a purée if they are heated gently with fructose or pure honey, to taste, and when soft liquidised or sieved.

Fruit purées are useful as an accompaniment to breakfast dishes. Alternatively, they can be frozen and eaten as a fruit sorbet or the juice may be strained off and used as a drink.

11

Footnote

It is some years now since I found my 'cure'. So what is life like now?

I am now in my fifties, menopausal, asthmatic, but NORMAL! My days are full, in fact there are not enough hours in the day to do all the things I want to.

Although I have not been employed for a number of years, that is not to say that I have been leading a life of leisure. In addition to all the normal work to which a housewife is subjected, our Springer spaniel dog Ollie was sick for several years and required constant attention. I also do Alan's typing, occasionally go out for lunch with friends, and do what I can to help others.

So, if anyone out there reading my little book is suffering as I once did, please don't despair; don't waste years of your life as I did. So much more is now known about food intolerance; the Exclusion Diet could be the answer to your problems. You have nothing to lose and everything to gain by obtaining medical advice on the subject.

12

Appendix

The *way* in which you record the details of your daily diet and how you are feeling, mentally as well as physically, is not so important as *what* you record. In a word, you should record everything. If you are in any doubt at all whether or not something is important, make a note of it. One thing is certain, if you think that you will remember it without writing it down, the chances are that you won't!

The following pages illustrate how I kept my own records and are included only as a suggestion of how you might like to keep yours. You may feel, however, that you prefer to devise some other method yourself or to buy a diary which devotes a full page for each day. The choice is yours, but remember that *everything* must be recorded.

DAY	TIME	DRUGS	FOOD/DRINK	SYMPTOMS
Weds	7:30 am	5mg Valium	Rice Krispies, Herbal tea	Panicky, racing pulse, indigestion, abdominal discomfort.
	10:00 am		Glass of water	
	11:00 am		Rice cakes, Grapes, margarine and banana, Apple juice.	
	1:00 pm		Salmon salad, Apple	
	2:00 pm		Pineapple chunks, Glass of water	"
	3:30 pm		Banana + pear, Apple juice	
	6:00 pm		Grilled chicken fillet, brown rice, carrots + broccoli, Herbal tea	"
	7:30 pm		Fruit juice	
	8:50 pm		Glass of water	"
	10:00 pm	5mg Valium	Herbal tea	Bed - feeling tired but still palpitations.

DAY	TIME	DRUGS	FOOD/DRINK	SYMPTOMS
Thurs	7.30am	5mg Valium	Rice cakes with Grarara, Mangarine & banana. Glass water	Panicky - feeling as I always do
	9.30am			
	11.00am		Homemade fruit salad: Pineapple, juice	Nasal discomfort and slight headache
	1.00pm		Tuna & salad Baked apple	
	3.00pm		Herbal tea	Headache much worse
	4.15pm		Glass water	
	5.30pm		Chicken, rice, green beans + carrots. Apple	
	6.00pm		Glass water	Headache becoming unbearable & I have never experienced anything like this before. Went to lie down as I was feeling very frightened that this headache would...

DAY	TIME	DRUGS	FOOD/DRINK	SYMPTOMS
Fri	7.30	5mg Valium	Rice Krispies with soya milk	Very relaxed last night. Headache gone. I feel different this morning - difficult to explain, not feeling panicky and abdominal discomfort has eased.
	8.30am		Green salad	Feeling totally relaxed and calm. In fact I can't believe that I haven't taken the car.
	11.00 am		Fruit salad, Apple juice	
	11.30am		Glass water	
	2.00pm		Grilled fish, rice & tomatoes, Pineapple juice	Completely panic free - actually walked to the shops and felt really relaxed. Really enjoyed walking round the shops. Quite feeling lucky to be able to walk out and get back home.
	3.30pm		Herbal tea	
	6.00pm		Banana	Still feeling relaxed. No indigestion etc.
	8.30pm	2mg Valium	Lamb chop, rice, broccoli & cauliflower, Baked apple, Apple juice	Reluctant to take Valium but decided to do so because I want to feed these new feelings as much as possible...
	10.30pm		Herbal tea	

Day	Time	Drugs	Food/Drink	Symptoms
Sat	8:00 am	5mg Valium	Rice cakes with banana margarine & banana	Still feeling very good, but standing to take Valium but must not leave them off until I ask doctor. Relaxed and well
	10:00 am		Glass water	
	11:00 am		Apple & pear pineapple juice	
	1:30 pm		Grilled fish & rice	Nasal discomfort, easing, I'm able to get a better breath
	3:00 pm		Glass water	
	4:00 pm		Fruit salad Herbal tea	Still feeling relaxed
	5:15 pm		Glass water	
	6:00 pm		Tuna salad Baked apple Pear Fruit juice	
	7:30 pm	2mg Valium	Glass water	
	10:00 pm		Herbal tea	Bed

DAY	TIME	DRUGS	FOOD/DRINK	SYMPTOMS
Sun	8.30am	5mg Valium	Rice krispies with soya milk	Feeling really good
	10.15am		Glass water	Haven't felt this calm & relaxed for years
	11.30am		Rice cakes & banana	
	1.30pm		Tuna salad Fruit salad	
	2.30pm		Glass water	
	3.30pm		Herbal tea	
	6.00pm		Chicken, new potato, broccoli & cauliflower. Baked apple	
	8.30pm	2mg Valium	Rice cake with Granose margarine	Missed my Sunday roast today
	10.30pm		Glass water	Still feeling very good — not even panicky.
				Bed

Notes

Notes

Notes

Notes